Living in

the Doctor's Nest

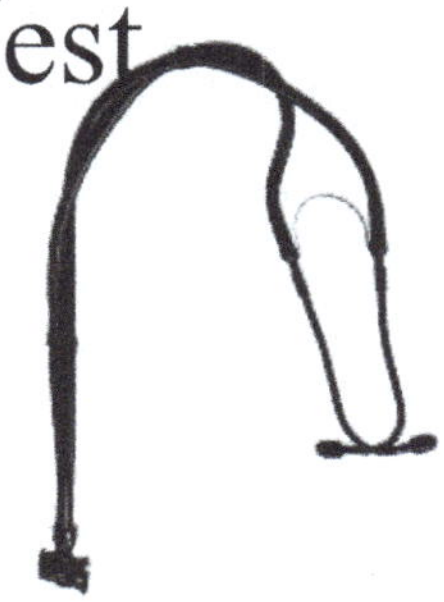

Anna-Karen Sorensen

Living in the Doctor's Nest

Contact:

aksorensen.com

https://www.instagram.com/theangelicpremie/
https://www.facebook.com/annakaren.sorensen.3
https://twitter.com/annakarensoren1

ISBN: 978-1-7330154-2-4

McKarr-Jonsson

Table of Contents

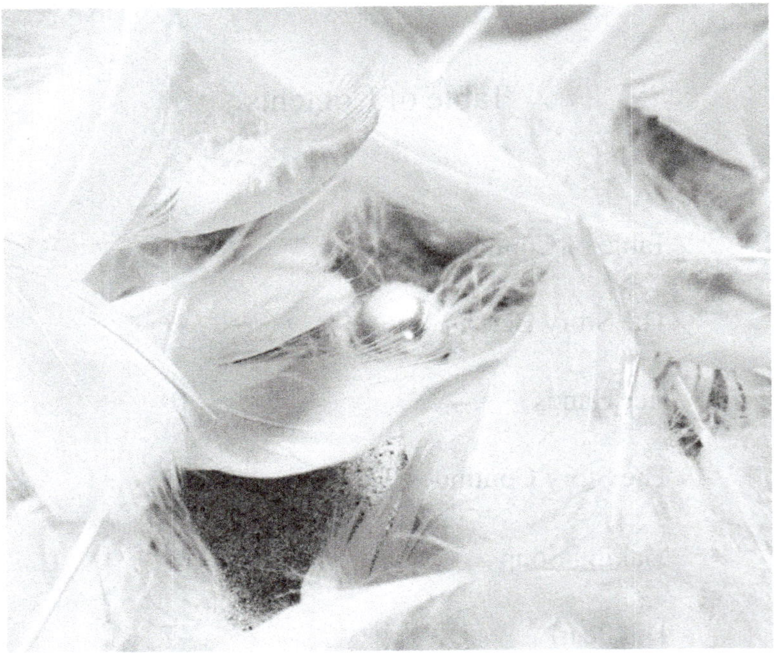

The cord of life both frees and binds
As flesh, it serves to sustain a life
As tether, it atrophies to naught
Leaving one in the world of strife.

It is no fulcrum around which to spin
Out of the world and out of place
Merely a leash that leads one from
The nebula into time and space.

The Story Begins...

Babies like to come that way, fast and in the middle of the night, at least the little ones seem to. It must have something to do with the silver light, and the angels, who on wing, escort them into time. So it was that I found myself driving in at 4 in the morning, splitting the darkness as I spirited myself into the hospital faster than could be humanly possible, or so I wished. There was never enough time, perhaps too little energy directed toward the tiniest babies and not enough science yet for the task that was needed to escort these little ones into time safely.

Tonight was just one night of many nights that had unspooled around the arrival of a new baby. It was just another event-filled and stress-laden bit of time that became the next pearl on the necklace of experiences that, strung together, became my life.

"Dr. Sorensen, they need you stat in L&D. They have a 27, or 28-weeker. She's at 9 cms and bulging. She's a walk-in," the voice on the other end of the phone announced.

I did not ask for more information but slipped my feet into my Ralph Lauren loafers, which at their stage in life were the leather version of threadbare. The loafers had come to the point on their timeline where I should have set them aside, but they were my lucky shoes, and I could not throw them away. We doctors and nurses are superstitious about things like that: about lucky shoes and jinxed beds, about full moons and statements that parents make in moments of pain or anger. Suffice it to say that we find safety in and cling to virtuous cycles and are reluctant to break them for fear of vicious turns.

Being continuously on call, covering the Pre-Q 24 hours a day, I usually slept in an outfit that I could wear into the hospital. My life needed to be efficient but also flexible, so clothes that could work for both day and night, and a mother who could fill in for me on a moment's notice made my chosen profession possible.

My life has been this way for many years, and I probably never have appreciated how completely the needs of the patients and their emergencies determined the path my life has taken. I have been involved with medicine in one way or another in school and training since I was 18 years old. I don't think I have known any other way of being in life as an adult. So it was that this night, as it was with many other nights, I put on my good luck shoes and headed to the green Jag. As I waited for the garage door to rise far enough for me slip out under it, I called my mother, and then I called the unit in that order to make arrangements for my children and to begin to set the plan of care for the infant that was coming. I gave the car a short voice command, "Call Mother," and it found my intended audience.

"Mom, I'm on my way in."

"OK," was all she said. I think her brain was trying to awaken, and that was all she could manage in the middle of the night. She understood what I meant.

The Jaguar had a phone in it, which was the first of its kind in the day. Although it is now commonplace to have a digital device attached to an ear or wrapped around a wrist, the car phone was a godsend for those of us who were on call. Without it, we would have had even less freedom to move about in our lives than we did.

While still on the phone with the unit, I started off for the hospital and drove around the massive white stucco house that sat sprawled at the entrance to our neighborhood. I eased my way past it and toward the traffic light. It was red, not surprisingly. I rarely caught it green. I slowed but did not stop as that light was a devil, rarely permitting me to proceed. Seeing no police, I moved past the eyesore and proceeded on through the intersection at a snail's pace, as though somehow going more slowly would help me evade detection. I made it past the light and out onto the highway, gaining some speed without being spotted, and I turned my attention away from the logistics of outmaneuvering obstacles and eyeballs to what was more important.

As I drove, adrenaline-pumped thoughts darted through my head, jacking my mind up into high gear. No matter how many years I had practiced Neonatology, it was always the same: I could not relax until I had the babe under control. With the birth of the early babies, it was as though I were standing in front of a large, dark tunnel with something that I could not see being thrown out at me. Perhaps it was the emotional residue of a recurring dream that I could not relate to consciously. This image was closer to the truth of the experience of being the caretaker of the premie than the analogy might indicate on first consideration.

You just never knew with these little ones. They had no back story, were not tested by life in any way, and had not proven they were serious about staying in the world. They just arrived, dropping their wings while falling into time, trying to die the minute they were born. We were given maybe 30 seconds to get them under control before we had to begin to worry about damage. They were born grey, wet and limp, and at this gestation, they were always quiet. Even if they tried to breathe, the tiniest of them could not move any air as their lungs were too stiff. With no air movement, they were silent even if they struggled, and if we did not get them supported quickly, they became still.

With this mother being a walk-in, I had even less of an idea of what to expect, not knowing what the condition of this baby was. I had not even heard if the mother was ruptured. I told the car to call the NICU as this baby, by its dates, was too big for the Pre-Q. The premie that is not micro, not being the otherworldly creature that is the tiniest of newborns, can tolerate the culture of the NICU. The tiniest of premies must go to the Pre-Q, which is a separate world that spins around its own center.

"NICU," the car answered.

With just that one brief exchange, I had a complete picture of the NICU staff member. It was Circi, who answered. She was one of the night nurses. I understood what she meant by her statements and what her talents were. She was one of those who hovered in the night, but did not hide in the darkness of it, which I found could be the case with night nurses in some centers. I was cautious about the nights anywhere else, but not here in the Pre-Q or NICU.

Circi had already called down to L&D to find out what she could, knowing that I would contact the unit on the way in. I was a good 12 minutes out, and after 30 seconds, I knew what she knew. The mother was 17 years old and had had no prenatal care. She came in with fever, and her membranes were ruptured. Circi did not know the mother's drug status, and the labs were still pending. The baby's heart rate and variability were good, but the fluid was cloudy.

"Who's down there?" I asked.

"Patti and Anna, they're setting up," she answered.

Anna was a nurse practitioner for neonates, an NNP. She lived closer to the hospital than I did and was a fast and sneaky driver, having lived in this town her whole life, she knew how to get through it without being stopped. Anna was my right hand, talented and dependable. I felt good knowing that she was already there in case I did not make it in time. Not arriving in time was the second of my repeated nightmare scenarios. The third was a real dream I had over and over of a baby extubating with no one seeming to care. It was difficult to discern sometimes where reality began, and the dreams ended.

When I arrived, I did not want to waste time hunting for the mother. Fewer nurses are on the schedule at night on wards, so I knew there might not be a nurse or clerk on the desk, and I did not want to find myself standing at the end of a long hallway with no idea where to go. Sometimes I used sounds to hone in as the mothers who walked in would have no medicine on board and no epidural, so I could follow the cries of pain to the correct room, but I did not want to risk that in this situation. The shorter the time since the admission of the mother, the less information we would have, and the more likely it would be that we might find ourselves dealing with a completely different delivery than was expected.

"What room is she in," I chirped, saving breath as though it were a limited entity.

"I don't know. I'll check and call you right back," Circi replied.

In the minute that was given to me, I called the house to make sure my mother had arrived. She had and was already back down in bed.

"The kids are fine," she assured me, allowing me literally and figuratively to push farther and further into the night.

The phone, nestled in the console surrounded by honey-colored gnarled wood, rang. It seemed out of place contrasted against the natural beauty of the console. I answered with a simple *yes*, long being out of the habit of answering calls with *hello* as they were almost always from the units, and formality at that point seemed ridiculous. Saying *hello* seemed rather like reintroducing myself in the middle of an ongoing conversation. As was the case with my greeting with a simple *yes* instead of *hello*, there was often no *goodbye,* just an *OK* or an order given to close out a communication. I spoke with the units throughout the day and during most nights, so being tethered to the units, my interaction with them was just one long exchange of ideas.

"She's in Room 6," Circi informed me and added, "She wants to push."

"Are they set up?" I asked.

"Yes, Ma'am," she answered in the formal way that was typical of the place and times. *Ma'am* was a title that was not commonly used where I grew up, but here it was, so I was always Dr. Sorensen or Ma'am. The whole of my tenure in the units, I was never referred to by my first name by anyone. It was a reflection of the understood responsibility that I bore. I was always on duty, ever the diligent guardian.

As I rushed through the last 5 minutes of the drive into the hospital, the asphalt whipped by, white lines compressing into dots as my eyes gazed at the black road that fell in the path of the headlights. I was always on high alert, watching for the police. No one would be on the roads at this hour in this sleepy town, and I would be noticed, and my speed assessed.

The police did not respect the existence of night emergencies, or that a doctor would be trying to get to the hospital quickly by dangling a stethoscope out of the car window as a clue. They used to let the doctors pass with this gesture, but it was no longer the case, so I had to be careful. I had to avoid being stopped and delayed, causing me to be late for the infant.

As I finished the drive, I thought about whether the baby would be a boy but hoped it was a girl. Girls did so much better; they were stronger than the little boys, especially as premies. A bit of stress also helped, as the lungs matured earlier and the babies could sometimes breathe at birth, even if they were very early. I could always hope.

Just then, the hospital came into view, and I winged around to the back and into the doctors' parking lot. I used my key to get in the back door and then pushed through the heavy double doors of L&D.

I heard the mother cry out once, already fed up with the pain of her labor. I was right, with this emergency, and with it happening in the night, there was no one on the desk. Everyone was in the back with this new mother and baby. I grabbed a gown and opened some gloves, size 6½, as I rushed down the hallway to the room from where I had heard the sound.

My eyes made the corner before my body did, and I could see Anna and Patti standing on each side of the warmer. It was quiet; everyone was still. There was no sound just then except for some whimpers from the mother. The obstetrician was sitting on one of two metal stools that were in the room, the other one placed in front of the resuscitation table waiting for me. In L&D, masks were not used, so I could see Anna and Patti smiling with relief that I had made it in time. I stepped up to the warmer.

"Everything set up?"

"Yes, Ma'am," Patty answered.

I could see the head crowning as I moved through the room. I preferred to check the equipment even though the staff was very competent, but there was no time this night. The baby was small and was delivering quickly. I tied my gown and put the stethoscope in my ears, tapped the bell to check it, and slid the stylet into the 3.0 ET tube, bending the end of it just a bit to hold its guide-wire in place, not letting it slip in too far and cause damage. I set the tube to the side on the clean field and rotated just in time to see the baby deliver.

Anna stepped forward with a sterile blanket, as the obstetrician handed her the baby. I stepped back to let her place the baby on the warmer, head down. We dried it quickly. It was a small girl that I doubted was more than 28 weeks. She was quiet, and we went about the business of drying. The baby responded and began to cry, weakly at first but then much more vigorously. The whole thing took less than 30 seconds, but those seconds seem like an hour when you are the one who is resuscitating.

I could finally relax, for when the babies breathe and pink up, we are well on our way. We did not spend much time in the delivery room in those days because the premies became chilled quickly by drafts and the evaporation of the amniotic fluid off of their skin. Added to that, they lost heat by conduction and through radiation as they tried to warm the walls and everything else that was around them. With the rules of thermodynamics applied, the babies always came out at a distinct disadvantage in the competition for heat. They cooled quickly in the cold rooms, and their outcomes could be dramatically altered by that stress.

About that time, Charlotte popped her head through the door of the delivery room. She was our newest nurse, just having finished the orientation program. Looking for action, Charlotte had headed down but was just a beat too late this time. We smiled, and she looked down, shaking her head. She knew, even with her brief experience, that if I was calm and smiling, then the baby was fine. If I was not attached to it, not bagging or hanging out of the side of a transporter, the baby was doing well. She headed back up to the NICU ahead of us, anxious to get some needed practice under close supervision as it was not the Pre-Q to which we were admitting the new baby. The Pre-Q was staffed only with the most talented and experienced RT's and RN's. The less experienced staff would work in the NICU for years before being allowed to take care of the tiniest premies.

Before heading up, and with the transporter ready to go, I took the baby over to the mother. She appeared distracted. No one was there with her. She looked at the baby only when I drew her attention to her new daughter. The mother seemed to be more concerned with what the obstetrician was doing. She did not want any more pain. She did not kiss her. She did not even touch the baby.

We went on up to the unit with Anna going up ahead, and Patti and I following some minutes behind. When we arrived, I knew something was amiss. The thoughts of the new premie, my concern with the mother's youth, and her indifference to her new daughter left my mind. I knew something was wrong in the Nest.

"What is it? Not a patient?" I asked as I paused my breathing.

I was reverting to a basic instinct that animals and small children use when they feel threatened. They become very quiet and quit breathing so they can hear better and sense more. Just as they do, I stopped breathing to better take in what I was going to hear.

"No, it's Anna. They just fired her and escorted out," was what I was told.

By then, it was 6:30, and the day shift was arriving. A buzz began to build as the news spread through the room. I sensed that the staff was not discussing patient information at that moment, but was mulling over the significance of what had just happened. Anna had been a significant presence in the units and an integral part of the Pre-Q, ensuring that it remained vital and that its energy stayed focused on its occupants. She put her life into protecting the units.

I had to stay and finish the admission, something with which Anna would have helped. When I had finished, I went up to the Pre-Q. Not addressing what had just happened, I rounded quietly by myself on the tiny babes, the under 27-week infants, who were its residents. As I moved through the unit, people tried to catch my attention. They all were aware of what had been going on for months. They wanted to see how I was going to react. They wanted to know what I was going to do.

I finished up and returned to the Jag. As I drove away, I spoke to the car.

"Call Anna."

Her Hands

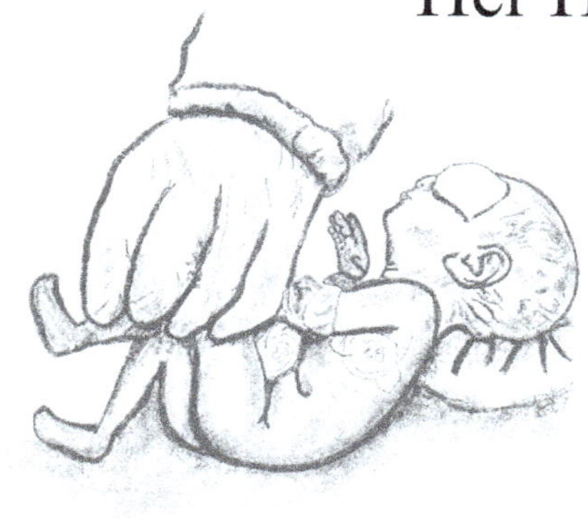

Bundled mummies are unfurled, and onto the tray, they are hurled. Papers rustle then are stilled as fine threads of hollow plastic, forced wet, are flushed of any bubble.

Flushed free of that fatal bubble
About which those not at the table
Care very little.

The arena shifts to hydrangea blue, and the field is illumined for a view. Sight is augmented with inky lenses as the deep sea diver leans in.

She leans in toward her keep
Taking care not to breathe
Avoiding any casual breach.

Encased in stretched synthetics, eel-like hands form the crèche that cradles and lifts the tiny babe. They position and constrain it, so it is made ready for its nest.

So it is made ready for its nest
Permitting her hands to do the rest
Of what is needed to attain their quest.

Needle thin pincers, as requested, probe to make the cord accept it,
the tiny lifeline that lies waiting to penetrate that space.

To penetrate that serpentine space
Which lies deep within the sacred place
Crimson flashes and is replaced.

Radiant heat on high does sear as its sensor seeks the veneer, any small piece of the thin-skinned one. To keep it safe, it must be baked.

The little one must be baked
Found by the sun through the gape
In the hydrangea colored drape.

She, of the hands, does suffer as sweat and lens mist do muster.
Muscle memory pushes through for speed in needed
so that progress can be made.

Speed is needed so that progress can be made
On the clock and on task she must stay
A thin line she must walk, disaster to evade.

Blue now gone, the seeds are sewn, and with time, its metal will be known. What hands can do has been done. The first hours carry so much weight.

The first hours carry so much weight
Say so much about the baby's fate
Does it have the strength to stay,

Orders are begun, tasks are done, and the moments begin to add up to a life. Nurses dart between intentions, as around the tiny one, we all do swirl.

Around the tiny one, we do swirl
As she sleeps and shapes into a tiny girl
Just a question mark she is before us, positioned in her gentle curl.

The babe is the ineffable become personal
The unknown, once rooted in the womb
Now cut free from its tether
To find its place in my world.

The Story Continues…

The baby from the last story was now a little "Borg," something like the character from Star Trek, no longer connected to the flesh of its mother by a pulsing cord but to the world through the humming wires of impersonal energy. It was doing well in the NICU, being small but not too small for that realm. It was big enough and strong enough to be able to bypass the nest that is the Pre-Q, so it was admitted straight into the NICU by me that first night without the help and support of my right hand, Anna. I had worked into the early morning hours on my own that night, doing double duty for that babe.

That was then, and so much has transpired since. Anna is no longer an employee of the hospital; she now works for me. The previous year, I had sent her back East to finish her training so she could become a neonatal nurse practitioner. Because she had been fired without cause, having become entangled in the exhausting power struggles meted out by the administration, I brought her onto my staff. Working in tandem again, she and I settled the feathers of the Pre-Q, and on the day that this next story takes place, we began to prepare for the arrival of a new 24-week premie. As it was coming so far before its time, it would not be admitted to the general NICU, but to the pre-Q to be taken care of by a select team that was committed to a small flock of premies for a month at a time. The Pre-Q would ferry this new babe across the river from its place outside of time to settle into a new rhythm with us.

Our homes, Anna's and mine, as we were both on a tour of duty in the Pre-Q this month, might need to be emptied of children on a moment's notice. Anna would drop her three kids at their father's, and I would take mine to my mother's if there was time, or if not, Mom would fly over to my house with a call. In spite of our efforts, we often failed to protect our families from the disruptions that medicine inflicted upon them. Anna and I had expected this lifestyle as we had chosen the profession, but our families had not and could not readily accept it.

Looking back now, I can see now how completely threaded through the tapestry of my life the demands of the units were. What I did not understand then, but now do, is how important the structure of the Pre-Q would become. It was not at all obvious that it would become necessary for a space to be created for the micro premies to keep them separate and safe from all else, safe from the rawness and aggression of the hospital as a whole and more specifically, from the clumsiness and distractions of those who did not have the touch for these fragile patients but did not choose to admit it. Over the years, as we struggled with many smaller moments, we would fail to appreciate the cost that this endeavor, the creation of a second womb for these most fragile of beings, would be to ourselves and our families.

At the time of this story, we were dealing with just one moment, not seeing the network of tissue that was growing around us. After rounding on both units and taking care of the practice that afternoon, there was still no 24-week baby, so I started for home. I popped back by the office, where I met my mother and gathered up both of the girls. They had a little playroom with a TV and a video player. Hope was still in a high-chair and had a playpen, and Perrin had a cute table and chair in the shape of a duck where she would play and eat. For napping, there were soft mats for the girls and a recliner for my mother, which she used between patients when she could, being the office nurse.

By the time we all got to the car, the sky had turned dark. I dreaded thinking about what the weather would be like by evening. The girls in their frilly dresses and matching socks and headbands and I, in something less girly, started for home in our shiny green carriage. We knew it would lose some its luster in the dust of the storm, and in the morning, I would have to try to stop Perron from finger writing on it. As soon as we arrived home, the girls shed their expensive and impractical outfits to grab some comfy pajamas, play with the dog, and have some dinner before bedtime.

The rest of the evening for me was peaceful if waiting for a starting gun to fire can ever be considered so. I practiced some French and took care of my personal communications as I had received only two calls from the Pre-Q. My favorite time of the day was the quiet time, the evening after I had finished my day's work, or had admitted a patient. It was during this time, the time of the late sun and sleepy heads, that I took a moment or two to reflect and to recover as I shook the day out of my mind. I stretched back in my chair, ate some dinner, and gazed out at the shades of nature through the bank of windows that formed the back of the house.

My backyard, hidden from the city by ten-foot cinderblock walls, had an honor guard of mulberry trees, one gnarled rain tree, and one very demanding palm. The palm tree was always communicating, tapping against the eaves of the house, reminding me of its presence. Less a watchdog than a greeter, Paris, my tall black poodle was invariably visible, waiting in her dog run. Whatever the weather, I could count on seeing her big black eyes searching longingly for a glimpse of us through the windows. She would walk as far as she could East in the dog run to keep us in her sites as we made our way between the two wings of the house.

Being home was a respite, perhaps more of a distraction, during which I could try to forget the reality of my life, which was that the work was never done. I knew there could be an admission or crisis at any time regardless of how many events had already transpired during the day. There was no such thing as a set limit. Still, on some level, I reveled in the break in intensity. Considering my tendency to take note of omens, I dreaded ever looking up to the sky and seeing a full moon during these times.

As we continued home, the weather worsened. I could smell the change in weather, as fine dust began to coat my sinuses. The sky had become an orange-tinted grey typical of the local tempests as the decay and dryness of the city whipped up into the air. To me, it was an ugly city and became only less so when it was snow-covered. It was a drab, barren, and uninspiring town and would have been tedious to drive through on the very first pass, but on later trips across it, it was just mind-numbing.

With the weather so bad, I decided to leave the car outside to avoid waking my children in the night if this hovering premie chose to drop its wings and fall. It was difficult to turn things off and let the day go as the atmosphere of the units drafted to my home, permeating every aspect of my life. I needed to force a shift in subject matter when I was away from the hospital, so I would turn on music from the BBC or some French movie on TV5, captured by the receiver of my one-ton satellite dish. To spice up my life, I ran copper wire the length of the roof to catch shortwave signals from Britain. I found any way I could to bring the outside world in, the world of culture and diversity, and shut out the monotony of this city. As I sat there, enjoying the respite, the phone rang.

"It's coming," is all the nurse said.

I found the Ralph Laurens and my purse and headed to the car outside. Its surface already resembled the dull rusted-out shell of an abandoned wreck more than it did the sleek, modern vehicle that it was, covered as it was with the soil of the city. I shut the door, and with the perfect timing that comes from years of teamwork, the car phone rang. Out of range of sleeping children, we made our plans. It was Anna, the night hawk who had flown across the city and landed in the nest, ready to take wing as she always was, energetic and prepared.

"I came on in. Bobby has the kids."

"How far along is it?" I asked.

"Only three cm's, but the variability is not good. I think they are planning to go ahead and take it. Everything is ready."

By the time I arrived at my destination, most of the burnt orange had blown off of the car, leaving it sadly dull, appearing uncared for. The car was often in this state, exposed to the dust bowl as it was. I made a significant effort to keep it clean. Still, it was hard to manage, just as it took a great deal of effort to extract a succulent life from this arid land. The area had only one thing going for it, the opportunity it offered to establish the units, the second wombs, in which the tiny babes could safely finish their gestations.

I had made this same trip, or a slight variation of it darting down some side street to change it up or speed it up, some 6000 times by my calculation, and I had long ago given up looking outside of the car for something to see. My eyes, as happens when one stares in the dark at a dimly lit object, began to see the city without distinct edges, as an endless sameness, just a negative space between my home and the units. Held in suspension during these trips, I pushed through them by filling my head with conversation or with music, depending upon the urgency of the moment.

The wind was still blowing when I arrived at the hospital, and as I leaned out of the car, my lungs filled with dust. I started to cough, not having planned the timing of my breathing well enough. Others were also arriving, hunched over and choking, gripping any barrier they could against the attitude of the city as they made their way inside. I was not alone in this struggle, but most who lived in the city had been raised there and had accepted it, not having made any decision about it. I saw what it was and had chosen it in spite of its atmosphere.

That atmosphere was dry, which was why I was drawn to my home with its rich earth, 50-year old mulberry trees, a well-established iris field, one gnarled rain tree, and that very busy palm. I bought the house for its privacy, the garden, and its palm, but the structure was a mess. The children of the original owner, not having had enough money themselves, had let it deteriorate.

Some fifty years earlier, there had been a pond near the back wall with spotlights over it and carp swimming in it. By the time I purchased the house, the area that had been decorative and vital, had become a quagmire of fish bodies and rotten leaves. The wires, through which light and energy had surged so many years ago, had transformed into wads of rust. I had to renovate the house before I could move in, replacing bullet-ridden glass, cracked pool decking, and disintegrating sidewalks, among many other things, all the while battling a well-established scorpion colony.

That was all before the arrival of the girls and the dog. Now it was my Oasis, a place that served to shut out the dryness and keep in the moisture needed to sustain the spirits of its inhabitants. The Pre-Q and the NICU were in their own way enclosed gardens, created to nourish the newborns, and as with my Oasis, they too had their brand of scorpions with which to deal. Short of killing ourselves in the house with poison or destroying the balance in the units with resentment, the scorpions could not be eradicated. We had to live with them, deal with them, and accept them as a challenge from which to learn and around which to move forward.

The crown jewel of the house was the bed of irises that ran 50 feet along the East wall of the yard, wrapping itself, serpentine-like, around the rain tree that would become my meditation space. The irises bloomed beautifully, although briefly each year and one year, apparently there were cycles, they served as the home for thousands of monarch butterflies. That year, I tried to capture their majesty on film as they danced and shimmered in the early morning mist that was thrown into the air by the sprinklers. It was a glorious sight to behold as the butteries navigated the blades, lighting on and lifting off of the violet bed, ensuring its future with their energy. I tried to capture that moment, but their speed and size made it difficult. Later, when I developed the photos, the butterflies, even with all their numbers and vigor, barely left any impression at all, but in my mind's eyes, I still could see their glory.

The backyard measured one acre with 20 old mulberry trees running the rim of it, only one of which was messy and fruity. Just as the iris bed had its seasons of monarchs, so the mulberry trees had their infestations of silkworms that covered the trees and everything near them. Luckily this did not happen every year, but it happened often enough that I had to paint the house every few years, which gave me an excuse to color the grey town with a different pastel shade of Florida each time.

My favorite spot in the yard was the bench that was situated beside the blood orange rain tree right in the middle of the garden within the garden, that iris bed. The locals called the wizened tree, a rain tree. As there was very little rain in the town and what moisture there was in the garden came from my sprinkler system, I did not understand why they gave it that name. The tree put out red leaves before the green ones, so it made a striking statement as it came back in the spring. My sacred place was bathed in a rainbow of colors, sometimes green and red, and other times, purple. When I was concerned about one patient or another, and I needed to reflect, to challenge my choices, or to listen to the voices of the patients in my head, I would find the irises and pause by the east wall, giving my spirit a chance to refresh.

In contrast to the calming effect of the iris bed, the palm tree was more of a distraction, a link to the blessed first decade of my childhood, to the coast of the south, the beaches, and my grandmother's house. Its presence would shift me emotionally to a time in my life that I remember fondly. Seeing that tree, I experienced a sense memory, a shift in my perspective rather than an anamnesis of any specific event or image. The fronds, with the sunlight dancing on and popping off, would startle my mind with their brilliance. The palm was an old southern tree that had no place being in this garden, but it had thrived by clinging to the house and utilizing that warmth to keep its juices flowing in the winter.

As it tapped against the eves, the palm would move like one of those windsocks that one sees along the road energized by a fan blowing air in pulses through it, so that it could catch the attention of the passersby. The palm's long thin trunk had years of trimmed fronds forming a collar that made it seem like a clown performing its act for an audience of one. I was never sure who the intended recipient of its efforts was.

Many things had drawn me to the house and had led me to see it as a sacred space, a place of support for me as I attempted to build safe havens for the premies. It began as a respite from the storm that was my life as an intensive care doctor on call 24 hours every day but matured into the sacred space within which the seeds of the second wombs for the infants germinated and grew.

All of us had to be as flexible as possible for me to succeed in my profession. We all had to bend our desires and twist our needs around the demands of the practice, for it was not the practice that would reshape itself to fit into our world. One way we could accomplish this was to arrange our days into 2-hour segments, selected to statistically increase the likelihood that tasks or experiences could be completed or realized. Living in fits and starts, those around me learned to protect themselves from the interruptions, to shield themselves emotionally from them, maybe even to deny them all together for they, especially the children, resented the demands that the Nests made on me and by extension, on them.

Living in the shadow of the Nests, we could not promise longterm commitments as there was almost no excuse that could be used to place my family's needs before those of the patients. My children knew it objectively, felt it deeply, and resented it. One night, when I had to take the girls to the hospital, Hope carved her name into the furniture where she had to wait for me. She made her feelings known that night, and ultimately, I had to unwind the attitude left in that room by replacing all of its wooden furniture.

With this new admission done, I returned to the car, the dust, and the trip back home. I felt my usual sense of satisfaction, having admitted a little one. Looking up, I could see the pale shell of the moon against the blue of the early morning sky, along with Lucifer, Aphrodite rising, set low. The moon looked lacy, just a sketch of itself, and although I was analyzing its potential for film capture as I often did, I could not help but note that it was full.

So it was at the end of this dust-filled day, I drove the car back into the gaping mouth of the house to enter the Oasis and escape the hostility of the city. So it was that I looked through the back window of the garage and saw my poodle, sitting with her black coat powdered with orange. She was waiting for me, as she did every night, with those sad eyes, half-covered with fur. She seemed to be begging to come in. As I think back, I lament the time she spent looking in at us from outside.

Even before I opened the car door, I could hear the palm tree tapping. The wind was still up, and the tap was more insistent than usual, so much so that I worried about the roof. The knock against the house was so strong that I could feel a vibration, something like the sensation that comes from an overexcited heart when it is driven by adrenaline, causing it to bang against the inner lining of the ribs. It is the same way that my heart pounds when I am about to receive a little one as it flies out of the darkness toward me, the sole provider, waiting nervously to catch it.

Before leaving the car, I asked it to call the Pre-Q once more to make sure everything was alright. In the seclusion of my office on wheels, everyone could remain asleep in the Oasis, undisturbed by the voices of medicine making late plans, attempting to put measures in place to retard the flow of calls during the night.

"Any change?" I asked in my usual succinct manner.

"No change," came the welcomed response.

And to bed I went, hoping for a few hours of dreamless sleep.

Making Soup

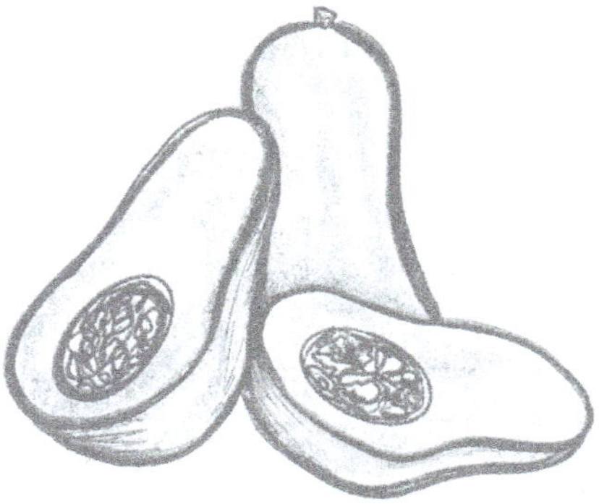

A day at home in the Oasis, which was miles away by land but only seconds away by thought from the units, was rare and often cut short. My life outside of the Pre-Q and NICU, the second wombs, was lived in a series of one-act plays. We had all settled, Mother, the girls and I, into a lifestyle that was less fluid by nature and more staccato in tempo, composed as it was of projects that could be interrupted, could be taken up again by me at another time, or at least could be finished by the others without my participation.

With time, my friends and family figured out that it would be safer to use two vehicles to attend any event. This meant there would be one chariot for my leap back to the hospital and to the babies during their emergencies and another vehicle for everyone else to use. In that way, those who were daring enough to spend time with me would be able to remain at the movie, concert, awards banquet, gymnastics competition or ballet recital, and experience the full impact of those moments. For me, as often and not, I had to take what I could get from the recounted tales of the events, living life through the eyes of others and wishing for more.

I do not remember any part of my adult life being any other way.

Being a physician, I was expected to be available to take care of my patients at any time of the day or night, in spite of my need for sleep or my family's dependence on me. I had to remain beyond reproach and be intellectually, physically, and emotionally available at all times. Because I had to prioritize my professional life over my personal time, my private life was stretched thin, often to the point of rupture. To equalize this great imbalance, I created something deeply sacred, and so the Oasis came into being. It was moist when the city was dry, quiet when the wind blew hard and vivid when the world was grey.

My life was lived in bits and pieces, in segments of 2 hours or less, with sleep experienced in sine waves, even on the calmest of nights, ebbing and flowing at the behest of the units, but not to the rhythm of my body. My projects outside of medicine came to fruition only if they could be subjected to some significant distortion, perhaps handled at an atypical pace, in multiple stages, or speedily. If something could be realized in 2 hours or less, it had a much greater chance of happening. That seemed to be a magical timespan, not too long, not too short, but just right for me to be given an opportunity to have a fuller life. Whether it had to do with distraction, accomplishment, enjoyment, or satisfaction, that space of time gave me room to breathe, to anticipate, and to experience.

So it was on the day of this story, I chose to make warm soup, one of my favorite two-hour endeavors. What a banal thing it sounds, but it is far from that. The experience of mingling with nature, of coalescing with it through the subtle intelligence of the senses, through vision, smell, touch, and taste, can become one of the *just-right* moments that realign the spirit, neutralizing some of the acid of everyday life. The act of creation distracts the mind from the awareness of the threat of intrusion: it puts consciousness to sleep.

Soup is liquid spice. Spice is the whiff that wafts us away from ourselves, out of the moment to another time. It moves us into a realm that is not understood through image or event but is felt as mood, the timbre of the era that existed when the spice first graced our lives.

Life is a process and is not static, it is creative by nature, realized through the overturn of the existent thought or event as it becomes the new idea or experience. Even when we do something simple, like making soup, we rescue the old and recycle it into something new. Soft corn and juicy apple meat join with the pungent juice of the cut onion. Feminine red mixes with regal gold and lively green as pulp and seed are transformed into a purée, and the house fills with the scent of oven-baked squash, as the ingredients shape-shift into a new experience within their cauldron.

As the soup's matrix dissolves within the boil, I balance on my suede ergonomic chair and maneuver an old heirloom bowl filled with washed green apples, dull apples, not the shiny ones that are treated to last forever, but apples that age naturally and become just what they need to be for my soup. I hold the blade of my knife at an acute angle and shave the skins of the apples away until just the sweet, but tart white meat is left. My fingers tire, but I keep paring until the flesh of the apples is exposed, and the old bowl has emptied into a new one that was purchased on a rare venture to an overseas port.

When I finish, I add them to the mix and sit back trying to stretch my back into a position that it does wish to take, my aching back, the back of my mother that has always limited my enjoyment of things. I reverse the bend in it and the pain lessons allowing me to go back under the spell of the soup. It is not only beautiful, sensual, and tasty, but it is virginal, free of the toxic salts and enhancers that so plague the world today. The purity of the moment assuages some of my angst over what we have done to the earth.

If there is no disruption, I deepen my joy by adding the rhythm of music. When the soup is done, its colors reveal themselves tinting the shards of autumn light, as they cut through the window glass of the Oasis. What could be more nourishing to the body and the spirit than to have the honor of being a witness to the ritual of creation and a participant in the shared experience of a warm cup of butternut squash soup?

As we all gather together, I take out the camera to capture some of the light: the golden rays of the sun, the dusky red shades of the leaves as they give up their season, and the rich harvest gold that is the soup's own glow. I try to capture the color before the grey of the world masks the moment. The color is too beautiful to shoot in black and white for nature does not show itself in shades of grey but rather, as the hues on the pages of life.

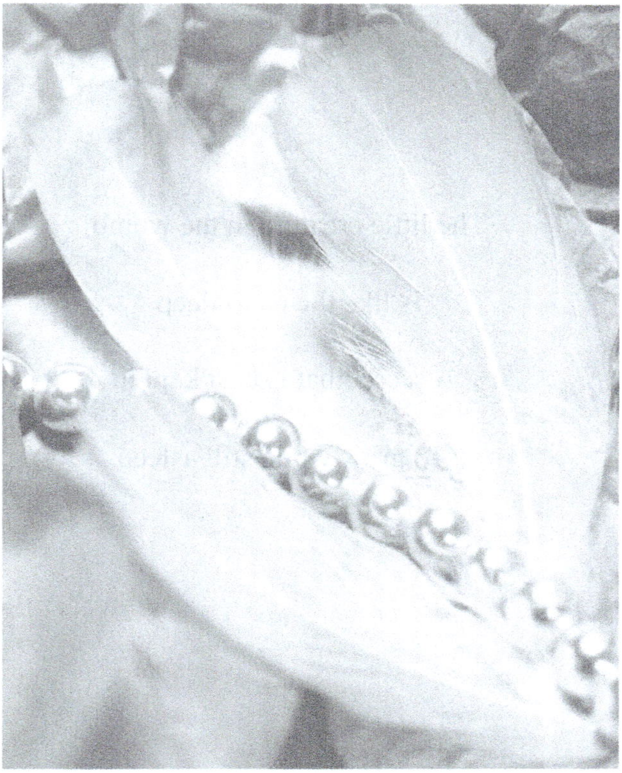

The little creature in the womb

Is like the pearl deep

A secret that is best kept in

To grow while still asleep.

The Pearl

"Ready?"

The obstetrician asked as he turned his head towards me, his body still facing the mother. He was looking directly at me at that point, so I just nodded, and with his arm in position, he entered her and pierced the membranes to expedite the delivery. As he readied himself to receive the head, the fluid gushed and then dwindled to a trickle. It quickly became evident that there was not going to be a little head presenting itself any time soon. It had not been the babe dilating the cervix but the bulging bag of water, and with the pressure gone, the cervix had closed back down. The baby returned to its semi-floating state like an astronaut in space, but with one big difference, this space was not expansive, but was shrinking and becoming more hostile with each passing minute. With these developments, I sat back and let the air leave my chest, a gesture something like sighing but with no sound. The pressure was off for the moment, figuratively and literally, but now we were in for a long wait.

As the baby was giving us some time, I got up and left the delivery room to talk to the charge nurse who was at the desk.

"Can you tell me anything about her?" I asked.

"She just walked in almost complete with intact membranes. She's not had prenatal care here. She denies any complications, but we don't have any records yet," she stated formally. "The mother did not seem to want to offer much information," the nurse added.

It appeared this patient would be a *tabla rasa*, a blank slate, a play that would be written in real-time with my team and me in active roles.

"She did say one interesting thing," the nurse said as she looked up from her notes. "She thought she was carrying twins."

"Anyone with her? I didn't see anyone in the delivery room."

"No, she's here alone. I don't know if anyone is on the way in."

While I was in the hallway gathering what history I could, the fetal strip had become less reassuring, so the obstetrician had decided to move the mother to the operating room in case an emergency cesarean section was needed. With the baby's head moving back in, and an unreassuring fetal strip, there was no time left for an ultrasound.

I shifted to the OR with everyone else. Newly papered from head to foot now, I sat down and let my back slump so I could push against the wall and give my scoliotic back some support. I had left my stethoscope dangling from my ears, so I would not have to touch the top of it at the time of the birth. I sat waiting, uncomfortable, but ready for what was to come.

The OR was a sterile place, or as lacking in character as could be managed. There was no odor, no scent that would indicate the presence of humanity. At best, it was medicinal. The walls were plain, free of any tint that could interfere with the assessment of the patient, and they were smooth, so they could be kept clean. They were also cold, and we lost our body heat radiating to them.

Trying to use my muscles to stay warm, I shifted on the stool using isometric movements to try to build up heat. I needed a distraction, so I addressed the team, which was still with me as I wanted a few moments to determine the state of things, and to decide who needed to stay and who should return to the units.

"Why don't you go back up and see if everything is ready in the Pre-Q?" I suggested.

"Yes, Ma'am," Patti replied as she turned to go.

She headed back up to the unit, filled with its micro premies who were still in the early stages of their lives outside of the womb. There was so much work to be done in this specialized space; every hand needed to be kept busy. With strict rules in place about who could care for these fragile little ones, there was no casual shifting of staff from here to there. With this being the case, the nurses and respiratory therapists did not call in for time off without good reason, as they had too much respect for each other and the babies. The only clear indication to call in for time off at the last minute was illness because the premie infant, being immune deficient, could not be exposed to infection.

With the pause, I shifted and pushed back against the wall again on my teetering, squeaky metal stool, a stool that was older than I was, I figured. Not much changed in the caverns that were the OR and L&D. When no one from the medical team was there, the cranky stool just rested quietly and was left in place, and when we were there, we were busy using it, so the distracting little seat ended up remaining, and I was made to sit uncomfortably on it, year after year.

Anna had stayed behind with me. We needed to assess the situation for a while before deciding to vacate the arena. She said nothing, as words were not necessary when what was happening was understood and anticipated. She just stood by the warmer, shifting her weight. Always moving, Anna was thin, athletic, and good with her hands. She was quick and impatient in general; she was about getting on with things. We all hated the wait and the lack of control, but it did not matter what we wanted to do, the babe would come when it decided to. We just had to wait.

I looked up at the simple clock with its shiny metal rim and big black hands circling in seconds, minutes, and hours, waiting to document the delivery time of the infant. My pupils, in saccade-like movements, returned again and again to the clock, but time seemed to be standing still.

Looking away from it and towards the surgical stands, I scanned the instruments that were lined up like tin soldiers, tarnished from years of use, anticipating this one last day of glory on the field. Just next to them, their disposable plastic replacements lay in waiting for their turn in the spotlight. In those days, these plastic instruments and wrappings were the new thing, and no one could have anticipated what this small gesture, this disposable product that seemed to be such a good idea and cost-efficient, would do to the ecology of the planet.

Just then, the L&D nurse caught my attention as she moved the light off of the mother. That light was the beacon that was necessary to have a good view of the procedures. It was bright like a sun but had the wavelength of the moon, which was more appropriate for this woman's experience in which we were all involved. No father was present and save for the obstetrician; it was all estrogen in the room.

The mother complained. The obstetrician snapped his gloves off in a reflex-like motion, a movement that he had perfected over the thousands of times he had put and on and peeled off the second skins.

“I’ll be in the lounge,” he said as he left.

He was probably going to watch television, some sports thing. We were, on the other hand, all stuck there in the arena. We were in a time warp in this now darkened, cold room with its walls made so slick in hopes that the bacteria would slide right off of them. It was a room with a floor that was hard and smooth, with no cracks, no grout to act as a refuge for the nasty things that could undo all the good we were trying to accomplish as we sat uncomfortably in our sterile garb. We were committed: gowned, capped, masked, and gloved. Even our shoes had paper covers over them. There was no way we would casually start over. No way would we throw away all that income. We just had to wait it out.

“At least there was no epidural to slow down the labor,” I thought.

It seemed to me, my mind responding to the non-verbal wisdom of my right brain, that things were a bit too quiet. No one seemed to be consoling the mother. No one seemed to be responding to her complaints as she moaned in pain.

My reflections shifted to the left side of my brain and to my life outside of the OR. As I ruminated over thoughts about sleep and not getting any and about handling the practice in the morning after this baby delivered, a pain suddenly shot up my back and forced me back into the moment. My back was rebelling against the circumstances that I had accepted as adequate, a cold room, a tiny unstable stool, and inadequate support. Contrary to what the textbooks had predicted, my back had hurt me since I was 12 years old, and it was not going to let me sit in peace on this night without reminding me that I was failing it.

I stood up with my arms folded across the front of my gown to avoid contamination and tried to use different muscles so the others could relax, and the spasm could subside. As mummified as I was, I still managed to stand up and rock back and forth, encouraging the dents in my female thighs to smooth out; marks caused by pressure against the metal rim of the stool that was made too small for a woman's anatomy, but just right for the male buttock. Like that stool, almost everything in medicine was tailored for the masculine mind and body, not for the feminine psyche and form.

I did appreciate one thing about this masculine footprint as I began my career in medicine. In contrast to nursing, which, as it expanded beyond its supportive role, filled out its degrees and job descriptions with wordy care plans and such, medicine, single-mindedly like Occam's razor, cut straight to the point.

Say what you mean and get on with it, was its implicit motto.

I appreciated that and could not tolerate meandering thought processes. The staff figured that out early in my tenure, and when calling me, especially in the night, they began with the bottom line, then retraced their steps to the explanations if I wanted more information.

As the night continued to play out in muffled tones, we shifted quietly but restlessly, generating soft rustling sounds and barely audible mumblings as we struggled to stay in formation. There was no tolerance for breaks in sterile technique, so appearances could become comical at times when one observed the dance of evasion that was undertaken to avoid contamination by falling objects or contact with the wrong side of another body. There was no effort ever made to catch something if it fell lower than the waist, just a lurching away from the falling threat. In spite of the awkward choreography at times, we were well-rehearsed, a fleshy machine made of components that ranged from the talented to the expert. We functioned by reflex and muscle memory, rather than by thought processes most of the time. All papered up and isolated from the patients, we stood at the ready, waiting impatiently for the night to move forward to its climax.

After another 30 minutes, I stood up and walked over to the warmer. I was cold as usual and stretched out my arms under the radiant heat. The stool just sat there waiting for my return, quiet now that I was not fidgeting on it. In those slow moments, it seemed as though my life had come to a stop. I stared at the black hands of the clock on the wall again, as though they would respond to the pressure of my fixed gaze and move faster in the way the crosswalk signal responds to compression of the button by the impatient walker trying to get the light to change. The clock did not care, the room remained cold, and my back continued to flare.

The mother moaned with each contraction. I shifted feet with each moan. I looked in her direction and noted that the paper drape that extended from beneath her and over the end of the delivery table had become heavy with amniotic fluid, resembling a splayed out tongue that was drooling and christening the pristine OR floor as it did.

Tarnished tools, slick bacteria-dodging walls, weary sluggish clocks, and a cluster of tired people all waited together. It was an odd welcoming committee for this new one.

The obstetrical nurse moved to the bottom of the table, slid her gloved hand into the mother, and located the head. The mother winced. The nurse did not. Something was different about the night.

"Who has the kids tonight?" I asked in hushed tones as I stood by the warmer. Nothing too personal was every discussed over the warmers.

"Bobby again," she answered as she shifted. "He was near."

"How is it going ?"

"One day at a time," was all she said as she looked back at the birthing scene.

I looked up at the clock again. That darn minute hand had hardly moved it seemed, but then neither had the little head. My mind drifted to thinking about my relationship with Anna. She had risked a great deal for me. Anna and I were closer than I was to the other nurses, she having been fired by the administrator because she chose medicine over the system. Because she worked for me now, we had a relationship that was more personal than were those I had with most of the other staff.

I had learned that in medicine, when one serves as the advocate for the patient who cannot speak for itself, it is best to remain as objective as possible so that when called upon to make the hard decisions, no emotional or political entanglements complicate things. For the units to work well, it required that the managers maintain some detachment; they needed to accept that their allegiance was to the babies first and to the sticky web of the social matrix second. In this way, they could remain objective enough to respond to the needs of the babies without feeling the pull of personal allegiances. When managers were reluctant to make this commitment, the units could be weaker. The nestlings needed to be guaranteed a safe place in which to thrive. We, who cared for the infants, had the responsibility to be available for and committed to them.

The mother moaned again, then she became more vocal. The obstetrician came back in to check her. I listened to the lowered frequency of the pulse being recorded by the fetal strip knowing what that meant. In the NICU and Pre-Q, as was the case in labor delivery, all of the monitors sounded out to the rooms. In this way, the caretakers could sense the status of the patient by the quality of those sounds. It is something I miss in the quiet units of today.

The units may be quieter now, but the babies are muffled and out of sight. They lie inside of quilt-covered isolettes, their courses un-witnessed, and the all-important feedback from the monitors is not processed through the subtle intelligence of the senses. The babes are isolated and hidden. I do not believe this way is better except to the extent that excess noise is kept under control.

It may be more comfortable for the practitioners of neonatology in these quiet units to hide in the computers in the next room, tallying up numbers, but the patient is left rudderless. These quiet units tend to function by consensus so that no one individual has to stand alone and take responsibility for the baby in the precise moments that events take place. Instead, the infant's measured values are passed electronically into a data bank to be casually reviewed as a summary at a later time.

The infant's data is viewed too much later to make the tiny adjustments necessary to avoid having to assault the patient with aggressive changes. This style of management leaves too few opportunities to make the subtle changes that are safe and timely. What used to be the practice of medicine has become protectionist, concerned more with legal exposure. What is prevalent in too many units is the safety net that consensus medicine is. It provides a hiding place for those who lack talent.

Just then, Patti popped her head back in. Experience had taught her that enough time had passed, and we should have had a baby one way or the other by then.

"Should I gown again?" she asked.

"Not yet," I said. "The head is not engaged."

With that, off she went back up to the Nest. All had been made ready in the Pre-Q for this little one who was young enough to gain entry into its sanctum. I could hope the baby was a girl, which would bode well for her survival and outcome. She was 24 weeks by her mother's dates, which is all we had to go by, not having an early ultrasound. That gestation was an early one, but one we could work with easily if all went as expected. I learned these few facts at the bed side as we waited, and had heard earlier that the baby had had a twin at some point, but they had found no second heartbeat.

Then the fetal heart rate slowed. It was dropping too often and for too long for this to be tolerated, but yet we waited. The situation was not reassuring and was coming to the point of being life-threatening, yet no section was called. We were locked in silence in the presence of the mother, so nothing more was said out loud.

Concerning extreme premies, a decision is usually made quickly, and either the baby is delivered vaginally or taken. Premies are at risk of being damaged during the trauma of vaginal delivery as they, unlike full-term infants, are not at the point in their development where they can tolerate the distortion of the skull and the drop in heart rate and blood pressure that comes with the process of birth.

The head finally came down, and I had Patti paged as Anna re-gloved. I unfolded the drapes, connected the suction, placed the stylet in the ET tube, and set the flow on the bag. As I moved to the side, I turned to the mother. Anna was standing with her hands folded across her chest, waiting for the obstetrician to hand her the infant.

The room had been low lit while we waited. Now the lights were back on, and we could see the head with its scalp in folds like a scrunched woolen blanket. Once it engaged, the baby, being so small, delivered quickly. It was passed to Anna. She stepped back and rotated, placing the infant on the warmer, head down. Without speaking, everyone did their part. Patti used her fingers to show me the heart rate as we briefly wiped the fluid from the skin, not so much to stimulate the baby, as to get it less slick, so we could work with it. The tiny body was put into position, and the ET tube was placed. Breath sounds were tested, and tape was placed around the tube and over the lip back to the temporal bone to anchor it. As heat is lost so quickly in those cold rooms, no lines were placed as she had resuscitated with ease. Instead, she was encased in sheets of polyethylene so she would not lose so much heat. As I bagged, Patti kept her finger moving to the rhythm of the heartbeat for me to see, and Anna listened to the lungs.

"Breath sounds equal and good," she said.

"OK, let's go."

With the plastic closed around the body and my hands anchoring the ET tube with two fingers on the tube itself and my palm and outer fingers around her head. We moved quickly to the transporter. An unplanned arrest was to be avoided, which could occur if the ET tube was dislodged or pushed too far into the trachea during the transport. I did not want to cause more stress for this little one, so we did not stop, but paused at the bedside trying to show the baby to her mother as we passed by her. She was preoccupied and did not notice.

Down the hallway, we flew with me hanging out of the doors of the transport unit like an appendage, bagging gently, never using too much pressure, feeling the compliance of the lungs with my hands on the soft anesthesia bag. It was hard for the micro premie to recover from the first few minutes of management if control had been lost by using preset ventilation protocols. With care, it was not necessary to give surfactant in the OR or DR, for with the rapid change in lung compliance that occurs with administration of surface-active materials and in the rush of stabilization, one can easily overestimate the force needed to ventilate the patient. If the patient did not come up easily and quickly with safe bagging, then sometimes surfactant had to be given early. Still, the cost of cold stress rose so rapidly with that maneuver that the risks had to be weighed carefully.

Anna had gone ahead to call upstairs while Patti and I followed behind.

“We're on our way,” she informed them.

As we flew through the doors to the Nest, we could see the team gathered around the baby's new home. There were new sterile trays and plastic ciphers but few tin soldiers. I was helped into a sterile gown, head cover, mask, and gloves. The Pre-Q nurses' trained hands quickly placed the baby, restrained it gently so it would not contaminate the field and adjusted the lighting. New setups were prepared, as the old ones in the delivery area had to be thrown away.

With the new IV tubes and stopcocks, care was taken to get all the air cleared. If the smallest amount of air crossed the foramen ovale, it could go to the brain. If the air bubble did not cross the foramen, it would continue straight through the right side of the heart to the lungs. Either way, air in the lines was life-threatening. Little bodies can not tolerate even the tiniest bubble.

With the equipment ready and the baby in place, we all moved into the field of action. Patti bagged gently as Anna dilated the umbilical artery, and I slid in the catheter into the abdomen of the infant and withdrew blood for a culture and a gas, clearing the arterial line of IV fluids to obtain an undiluted sample. I then slowly replaced the expressed blood.

A second line was placed through the umbilical vein, this one traversing the liver, which could be tricky for as the oxygen tension rises in the blood, the path closes quickly, and the catheter sometimes does not pass through to the heart. There was a maneuver that could be used to get it to follow the vein. Out the line would come, and with pickups, I would twirl the end of the catheter around the metal tips of the forceps, forcing the catheter to curl ever so slightly and temporarily but just enough so that I could spin it and tweak it through the closing duct.

"We're through," I said as I tickled the walls of the atrium with the tip of the catheter, giving the patient a brief dysrhythmia. It was verification without the x-ray that we were through to the heart. The catheters were taped loosely in place to be anchored later using protective skin after their positions were understood. Then Anna and I stepped back, arms crossed in front of us, as always, in line formation. The X-ray machine moved in, and a shot was taken to make sure the line placement was safe before we pushed any fluids. We administered or replaced fluids very cautiously, and in small quantities, everything with these tiny ones was done in small steps by gentle hands, always with attention to detail.

Then we waited, but by this time, I was usually overheated and sweating. My skin could not breathe under the latex and paper scrubs as the heat was overwhelming under the warmer. The tiny premie has a small surface for the radiant warmer to find, and once we cover it with drapes, the warmer cycles on frequently. We must be baked so the baby can stay safe. The baby must maintain its core temperature, or it can succumb to a cascade of coagulation issues.

While we waited, the surfactant was drawn up. Before the availability of surfactant, which I worked on isolating in my research, we could only hope to save babies down through 25 weeks of gestation. With surfactant, we could successfully work with babies down through 23 weeks. The 24-week gestation infants with exogenous surfactant on board were good babies to work with, and without unusual circumstances, did very well.

With experienced providers, the lungs did not need to be damaged.

With talented hands, the lungs and the provider worked as a unit and the person who was bagging adjusted appropriately. The inspiratory time was kept short to avoid becoming trapped in a cycle of damage. Patty was bagging while I was still in sterile garb, so both she and I became very hot. Anna was working on the orders and was cooling down. I could feel the moisture collecting in my gloves. Just in time, it would seem the Xray would arrive and be put up on the screen.

"Good placement," I said as I stepped back and peeled off the layers of insulation as fast as I could so my body could breathe again. I retreated to the staff break room, which had begun as my office but had become a gift to the unit. I sat down as Mere, the baby's new nurse, connected the umbilical lines to the IVs fluids, and set the drip rate based on the baby's size and gestation. There were fluids of dilute salt and fluids with glucose and electrolytes for the baby's lines, always with heparin to keep clotting at bay.

Next, the patient was released from its constraints and placed in a fetal position to try to recreate the intrauterine environment. Her eyes were covered, and she was sealed into a tented plastic enclosure to decrease fluid losses and create an environment that was not hostile for her. Consistency of humidity was of paramount importance with the tiny ones, as they lost so much fluid straight through their skin that it collected on the sides of the plastic tents that surrounded them, forming droplets. Erratic fluid control could result in poor management and life-threatening interventions.

After the storm settled, the area around the babe became quiet. I looked down at her without the stress of the arrest that accompanies the birth of the tiniest ones. I could see the babe as a little being rather than as a crisis, could appreciate the gentle nature of her presence.

With the ventilator carefully set, based on the gases, X-ray, and clinical exam, Patti could rest her tired hands and let the machine do the work. When I first started in medicine, I did not realize how close to the beginning of the specialty the times were. It had not been many years before I began to train that all babies who could not breathe on their own had died. Now a few generations of ventilators later, it was possible to trust the machines to do what we set them to do, but we still had to be vigilant.

Even now, we needed to remain focused on the patient, for just as the baby had quickly adjusted her ventilation needs post surfactant, so during the next hours, the compliance of the lungs would deteriorate again, and she would require more support. This was expected and could be managed if there was someone who understood the phenomenon. This short period of stability was called the honeymoon phase. It was the time when the patient could proceed under full sail, with lower positive pressures needed to ventilate as long as she could continue participating effectively, as it required not only compliant lungs but consistent effort.

After the honeymoon phase, the lungs would stiffen again, and the air movement would decrease as her bellows became less compliant again. At that point, we would move in and assess, following her lead as she indicated to us how much support she needed. For the moment, this patient was in the early stages of her honeymoon, so we had some hours of relative calm to enjoy.

I looked down at the little thing again. She was soft, with beautiful skin that was translucent with pores so tiny, they could not be seen with the naked eye and a face that was less pretty than it was fetal. The baby was cute at this age, but soon with the mobilization of some of her body fluids, she would begin to look like a very wizened 95-year old man with chin fuzz. It was a sign of health that the patient mobilized its extra fluids. At this point, this new little one was still smooth and silky.

In the morning, we would do an ultrasound of the brain to look for any evidence of capillary leakage, the second most important predictor of the future well being for this child, with the first being the quality of the lungs. After I finished up, I finally went back down to talk to L&D. I needed whatever records they had put together on the mother. Having been there through her birth, I knew what the baby had gone through during the last hours, but I needed more of the maternal history. I caught one of the night shift nurses as she was leaving. Raising my shoulders, I looked at her quixotically. What she answered to my gesture, I had never heard before.

"She did not want the baby," the nurse said, looking into my eyes.

"She would not agree to a section," she added. The obstetrician could not do a thing with her, and the baby was in trouble, but he could not get her to change her mind."

I had sensed that something was not right. It seemed like everyone was going through the motions, but with a different air of expectation. There had been no joy in the room.

The nurse spoke again, "the obstetrician was quite upset. He had never had a mother refuse a section when the baby was in trouble."

The nursing staff knew the mother was indifferent to the baby, but it still surprised them. Most of them, being mothers, could not understand it.

“Everyone felt sorry for the baby. We had expected it to die,” she added as she turned to leave.

I turned my attention to the chart to find the information I needed and then went back up to the Pre-Q and let the staff know that the mother would not be visiting the baby that night. Usually, on the way to her room, a mother would be rolled into the unit so she could see her infant. General anesthesia and surgical closure could delay this at times, but the visit was not going to happen with this babe at all.

After that, I left to get a few hours of sleep before doing my morning rounds. Anna had gone on home relieving her ex, but Patti was there for the night.

The morning arrived the instant my head hit the pillow, just a moment it seemed after I called the Pre-Q one more time to discuss the labs, vital signs, and gases. By the time I got to the unit in the morning, the ultrasound technician was setting up. The baby had done very well during the brief time she had been with us. It was a bit early to look at the head, but the study would still give us some information if there was a significant bleed beginning.

Walking over to the baby's bed, I glanced over the shoulder of the technician as she placed the sensor over the anterior fontanel, a window into the brain in the very early born, and made a wide sweep to get her bearings. I glanced at the screen as she began the study and then looked down at the probe for some explanation of what I saw. The technician was also challenging herself, changing the angle of the probe aggressively, assuming there was something she could do to change the image. I stood there for a while as she maneuvered, and then I spoke.

“Is it what it appears to be?”

She just nodded as though with this kind of situation, one should not say anything out loud. The study showed that the brain, down to the basal ganglia, had been replaced with fluid. The little thing that had appeared so healthy and had acted so well during the first hours of life was functioning on its primitive brain and brain stem. She had no mind, no cortex with which to think.

I sat down, feeling betrayed by science, feeling entirely impotent. There was nothing more I could do for this babe. I could not wish her well. There was no medical trick that I could use to give this little one a future.

As I sat there, I wondered what role the hostile environment had played in this. It was not scientific to think that there was any connection, but the truth could not be denied. The babe had not been wanted, and she had chosen, as had her twin, to go away.

So it seemed in the end that....

This little creature in the womb

Unlike the pearl deep

Was not a secret best kept in

To grow while still asleep.

Coming Next: Short story #5

"The Boyfriend"

Made in the USA
Monee, IL
04 November 2026

67382293R00046